HOW TO FINALLY LOSE SOME F*CKING WEIGHT

By Richard S. Roy

HOW TO FINALLY LOSE SOME F*CKING WEIGHT

By Richard S. Roy

TABLE OF CONTENTS

For Goldy, Jerry, DJ, Rose Demetrius (grandma), Nabu, Javyn, Jeremiah & my closest friends.

"For the best parts of me, reside in my friends and family."

"Vivre une vie epanouie devrait, etre votre seul desir."

Foreword

"Struggle is evolution." A phrase that popped into mind as I was struggling to bring the Browns home (Ironic) to the super-bowl. The idea that brought both of those thoughts together is how struggle a) takes place in a myriad of ways, and b) struggle doesn't always produce favorable results. In fact, most of the time we succumb to our downfalls! However, this is not to say that struggle is not a critical component to our ever-evolving self. How do you suppose we got to where we are right now?

Regardless of how you feel about the current life and times, this is the most prosperous age of our species' genealogy. How does this come together in a weight loss - self-help book? It does and it doesn't. In short (and you could probably put this down or turn it off after acknowledging this segment) fitness & nutrition do not have to be a struggle. Living your best life doesn't have to be hard & a clear mind shouldn't be a challenge for these things are entitled to us in regards that we each hold the capacity to attain what we truly desire. Is there an element of "struggle" & work? Of course, this is where the duality takes place.

At the end of this book you'll learn how to put together a workout program that works for YOU. We'll explore different strategies and give you the tools you need to make a decision that works for YOU using the facts and modern scientific research. You'll learn from my struggles and in turn help motivate someone from your very own. Today, we're going to learn how to finally lose some f*cking weight.

Chapter 1 - For the Love of Fitness?

So, who the hell am I, & what warrants me the right to write a self-help book based on weight loss? Fair gumption. My name is Richard Roy. I am Founder, CEO & Head Coach of Scintilla PT. We are a Personal Training service that specializes in custom high quality personal training for all individuals, without breaking the bank. It wasn't always this way, however. I come from a background of both Big Box, & Corporate Personal Training. Being certified for a decade, my career started very early. My story is a long one, & the details do not fit in this book, but allow me to paint a picture for you in hopes you can understand my perspective, & why I do what I do.

The year is 1993. A young legend was born. Born in New York, from Haitian immigrant parents. My father was out of the picture by the time I was one year old. My mother, Goldy raised me & my two brothers herself, along with the help of my grandma, Rose. My mother's story is also an odyssey but that is for another book perhaps. Even with the hard times, we still managed well. My mother wasn't the type to ask for handouts and always preached resiliency & faith in God, so for the family & I, everything was pretty cohesive. For the exception of my brother DJ. He was the middle child. He was a self-proclaimed "genius" who was born in Colombia & made it to America with my mother and brother years later. Growing up he was very popular but ended up running with the wrong crowd later in his high-school years. But he managed to curtail his behavior for the most part, & becoming a better role model for me, & what ensued was a great relationship between my brother & I. Always giving me advice when he could & told me his mistakes in hopes I would avoid them when he couldn't.

My mother used to work nights. Some nights when she would leave for work my grandmother would be on duty. Like the amazing grandmother she was, Rose would stay up all night making tons of fried foods & pastries. Dj & Jerry worked at Ralph's pizzeria in Staten Island. We lived two blocks away so every night they would also bring food. Imagine this; a twelve-year-old, eating calzones, washing it down with soda, hanging out with his older brothers playing Mario kart at three am on a school night. Pretty sure that's every kid's dream growing up. Eating whatever, whenever. The experience served in more ways than one. For starters, its increased bonding time between my grandmother, brothers and I. Growing up getting to hang out with them was always the highlight of my day. Even when we were all on bad terms. The trio was inseparable, & I was the little tike running behind trying to catch up. Rose was in on the action too! The second lesson was, I got fat, fast.

'til this day if you ask my mom, she'll still complain about how hard it was to find clothing in my size growing up. At 13 years old I was roughly 210lbs and heading in the severely wrong direction. Now my brother Jerry played High School football for Port Richmond and had graduated pretty recently, but stayed home because he fell in love, as opposed to following his football dream. I love my nephew & ex sister-in-law so no hard feelings there. However, in between his career limbo, he wanted to teach me everything he knew about football before I got into high school. I always wanted to play but we couldn't afford to play in the private leagues outside of school, so we chose the academic route. I was stuck playing basketball for a Catholic church basketball program called Upward instead.

It was a rainy summer day. Junior High had just ended & I was a staggering two hundred twenty pounds. But I had running back dreams and hands that could catch anvils, so I was willing to do anything. My brother Jerry had the grand ole idea of playing tackle on the cement in the busy intersection across the street from our house. We had an event called the Big Apple Games coming up later in the summer, it was for all the high school football teams on the island and he wanted me to be ready for it. The intent was there but boy, did that fucking backfire, hard. Jerry positions me on the other side of the street. No cars coming from either direction. It was still early, and the rain was coming down pretty heavy, as if this was a scene from *The Chocolate War*. Except without the Vigils and other antagonists. Raindrops striking his furrowed brow, he looked at me with a stern look on his face, like a Sergeant addressing his soldiers before storming Normandy and said to me "Richie, I'm going to throw the ball to you like it was a kick return. "I want you to run back to me and just practice taking a hit. Ok?" "Ok." I replied, as I swallowed the air in my throat from after stammering to oblige to what already felt like impending doom. You know those moments when you can tell something is going to go wrong? I believe that is what they call *"intuition.?"* This was one of those moments.

He throws the ball my way. Again, I have magnets for hands, so my first fatal flaw was catching the damn thing. But most importantly, listening to my brother when I should have listened to myself instead and had **stayed within my limits** of practice. In other words, why was I practicing with someone who was at a collegiate level, when I was an incoming freshman? Loyalty and lack of resources make you do creatively disastrous things. After catching the ball, I immediately make a b-line for the other end. I figure If I run faster than him, I can definitely avoid his hit. Wrong. This man threw his body at me. He hit me like I *wasn't* family. Me and my brothers had different fathers and I knew, but with that hit Jerry let me *know*. I'm looking forward to the day we can insert memes into books because this certainly deserves one. After the initial hit, I stumbled but managed to keep balance until I took another step this time with my left and it slipped from underneath me. The result of that was not the cool Rick James split but more so of the "oh my god, I should probably go to the hospital to fix my leg because I can't move it" variety.

A jolt of intense pain shot up through my hip like an electric shock from a live powerline if you were too close. Heat from my hip joint itself grew in intensity and my leg lay there in a position so unnatural to human anatomy you would have thought I got struck by a Durango.

After wincing and screaming in excruciating pain, my brother helped me up and brought me inside. Everyone in the house surrounded me, like tribal villagers onlooking helplessly as a fellow member succumbs to an unknown poison & the Shaman tries to heal him. In this case the shaman being my mother. She was seemingly trying to diagnose me without knowing a lick of medicine. But just like most foreign households, we often revert to "house medicine" as I call it before we do anything drastic like see a *health professional*.

My mother thought I had pulled a muscle… & we found that was definitely wrong. But I haven't gone to the hospital just yet. My grandmother lathered my leg with Vicks Vapor Rub & we both agreed that was all for now. The pain had subsided, but I was in for a severe awakening.

A week or two go by & although I cannot run full speed, I have a little pep in my step so I can make short receptions & tip toe out of bounds. That's what me and my brother worked on. Every movement hurt but considering I didn't want to let my brother down I pressed on. When we finally make it to the BAG. They had the skills position players line up first for warm up drills. Skills positions are the players that get the most contact with the ball or potential too, outside of the Quarterback. These are your Running Backs, Wide Receivers, Corner Backs, Linebackers etc. I made my way over to the Running Back section & that's when all hell broke loose.

First drill was a basic lunge. And that exposed the integrity of my hip joint indefinitely. The second I took a step into that lunge, immediately I felt the joint fully give way & pop not only out of socket but break in the process. I hit the floor with almost the same velocity & speed the first meteorite did that met the Dinosaurs on that fateful day. Coaches came equipped with a wheelchair and I was sent to the hospital for x rays. I had a displaced hip joint with a hairline fracture going through. I required surgery, and at that moment both my football dreams, and my summer were over at an instant. A hip injury is bad news for any football career. This I could say was my first encounter with struggle. But it certainly wouldn't be my last either.

May 3rd, 2011. A day for me that will forever live in infamy. To keep this a self-help book & not an autobiography (soon come) I will fast forward the story that is my life. It's now Senior year of my high school career. I'm a full blown "skater" (bye - bye football) My leg has made a full recovery & I'm a happy healthy teenage boy. Finally starting to get noticed by females (by way of my newly found physique and confidence) becoming more popular and becoming more social. Life seemed like it was on the up and up and nothing could bring me down. I even had good grades for the surprising amount of times I was cutting school. I would leave after main attendance to either skate, or hangout and play Halo with my friends Paul, Chris and John. My friend Andrew was the special guest star. He didn't skateboard but loved video games as much as us if not more, and he lived on the same block, so it worked very well.

It was May 2nd, about 7pm in the evening. Just the night before Doomsday. My brother Dj had just gotten home & at that moment in time we weren't on speaking terms because I ate his sandwich. Petty, I know, but imagine if your little brother ate your food over and over, regardless of the warnings you gave? I was coined the nickname "Human Waste Basket" because of my eating habits. Funny & a bit shameful? But I digress...

I step out the door, making my way outside. I had plans to meet with my friends that evening for some good ole Halo action. The second I stepped out I bumped into my brother. "Yo." DJ murmured. He was dressed in work clothes, but he had a slight smell of alcohol on his breath. Happy hour must've been fun. "Yo...are you still mad at me?" I whimpered. I loved being on good terms with my brothers because we were so close, so if any of us had an issue, at some point we'd make it right. "No bro, I was just stoned and hungry that's all. Don't worry about it." He chuckled. Dj was short fused but always came to his senses. Often apologizing even if he wasn't in the wrong.

We hugged and I asked him where he was going that night. He mentioned he was going to the studio (which wasn't in the best side of town) to finish a track he was working on. At the time he was working on a new track for his upcoming debut album. Indie artists were able to put their own music on Apple iTunes so it was finally his time for the world to hear it. Unfortunately, I didn't know that would be the last time I ever see my brother again. The silver lining is the pain from this tragedy inspired me and turned what used to be a hobby between me and my brother into a full-fledged service, dedicated on inspiring and helping others. But this is also where I truly began to learn the meaning of struggle, depression & exactly what kind of demons that can plague the mind during times of crisis. Although we can truly never know what will happen in life & can never fully control the external circumstances outside of personal choice, we can control one thing. The mind.

The biggest takeaway I want you to have outside of your revenge body that your ex will soon drool over is how to use your mind. No, not for just thinking & common sense. How to use it to visualize your dreams, visualize your future, visualize what the already perfect version of you looks like, but match that with work to make it come true in its physical manifestation, not just your head. In closing of this chapter, I want to leave you with a thought before we dive deeper into the world of fitness;

When you think about a seed, or the transformation of it. Typically, at its simplest form, a seed simply needs sun, soil, & water. Right? But the seed itself inherently, is just a seed. Now built within this seed it already has the necessary ingredients to grow to its fullest potential. Water, sun & soil are mere catalysts that support the growth of said seed.

You begin the gardening process, and after some time goes by, you finally have your flower. You knew what the outcome was going to be before you saw the final product. You stayed the course and saw it through and as result it had to grow. Even when you saw nothing you did not waiver because you followed the process and stayed true to the vision of the birth of that flower. Now, let's say we are this seed. If our mind is the soil, words the water, and action the sun, what If we "planted" ourselves in the faith that we can make it to our destination and manifest our innermost desires?

Using our imagination, what if we pictured in our mind what our newly improved self would look, talk and act like? Would we not follow the course if we already knew the result? This is how your mind works. It must follow suit and physically manifest anything you think about a majority of the time. Does this mean you'll manifest 1 million dollars in your bank account? Of course not. However, who's to say that if you felt in your heart and soul that you were a millionaire and had something of value to give the world, and that was your core belief, your predominant thought, would your actions not follow suit and find ways to become said millionaire by finding a way to help others around you?

Let me ask it another way. If you knew in your heart & soul you could finally lose the weight, get in the best shape possible and live life fully untethered, would your mind not look for ways and strategies to achieve that? Here's the truth: whether you're doing well in life or subpar, in some form or another that is all your own doing. How you react to your circumstances are ultimately what shape you and this also rings true for your daily habits whether that be action or thought, because your thoughts are what precede your actions.

So, without further ado, let's start the show.

Chapter 2 - Get your mind right

Between 2011 and 2019 I've lost my grandmother and my second brother. I've contemplated suicide and even attempted it. I've been fired from a position I was utterly devoted to, to delivering pizza. Only to get another job as a coach, to be fired a year later from that one as well. I've lost a relationship with someone whom I thought I'd spend the rest of my life with, but fortunately fate had other plans.

We spend countless hours attempting to please other people, even when we know ourselves that we don't want to or rather, have something of our own we need to accomplish. Putting it to the side and compartmentalizing what is paramount to us as secondary to someone else's needs. Am I telling you to be selfish? Yes. But not in the way you may be thinking or already know in regard to this topic. I do believe there is a case to be made here about being selfish, and I'll stake my claim now.

During my 10 years of being a coach, I've had dozens of clients cast off their own fitness goals because a spouse had the demand of making a certain food or eating a certain way because they themselves were not ready to make such a change. Even though the obvious outcome would be a very positive experience and not only life changing for the person specifically on their weight loss journey, but as consequence beneficial for both parties. From my experience I've coached couples together and they have made long lasting changes. On the other hand, I've coached people to make 180-degree changes in their life… only to toil away their hard-earned efforts because of the lack of support in the home. Growing up, my mother always instructed me on one thing when it came to relationships. "Make sure your partner supports your positive endeavors & can be critical of the negative ones for you both will be affected by each other's actions, & reactions." I still keep that in mind 'til this very day.

The mind is a funny thing. It hates growth but demands it. It hates complacency but feels safest in the clutches of normalcy. It ridicules you for staying still but compromises your morale when you begin to move. Why are we built this way? These ways are mainly predicated by environment, influence, and past experiences coated in a slew of genetic code predisposing you to success or failure by what you see, feel, & hear. Everyone on this earth is capable of living their wildest dreams but it is only those that work to achieve the ideal that truly see Valhalla personified. In other words; yes, your spouse & or environment may be weighing you down. Hopefully not down for the count.

They say the mind is a terrible thing to waste. I'd agree & also disagree. You see, there is no real "wasting" of time or mind. You're simply allocating your energy to something else, something easy. Unfortunately, in today's day & age being distracted is easier than ever. Not necessarily through our own fault sometimes, the silver lining here is that most of these applications on your phone are designed specifically to be attention grabbing. I mean, the goal is usage at the end of the day… & I'm sure you may have a new selfie you want to add onto your profile. However, we cannot be blind to the facts & deny the binds that we ourselves tie because of that one feeling every human innately has. What is it you ask? It's fear. Fear of what? Who could possibly be afraid of getting healthier?

You'd be very surprised. It's not the health aspect that would scare someone, but more so the idea that they would have to make long lasting changes that could potentially affect nearly every crevice of their life, & it will. It has too. It should. Hence why it is a change. You are exchanging your former self, your bad habits, intrusive & negative thoughts in place for something that may seem greater than you now, but when you achieve, you'll come to realize that it was rightfully yours the entire time. This is exactly how all things in life work. There must be a sacrifice. There is never nothing for something. Nothing is ever free in this world & that is okay.

Let me ask you something, when was the last time you truly cherished something that was for free? Never. If you did, you're an outlier which is an anomaly in recurrence. Humans are built to take things for granted & consumption, or that is how society has deemed us to be. We all still have the choice to take the other path. What is the other path? The other path would be the realization that you truly deserve more in your life & solely you are holding yourself back when it comes to achieving what you truly want in this lifetime.

Without going deep into the spiritual rabbit hole, we don't know if there is an afterlife or if you get a chance to redo this when this is all over. Why wonder what could've been? Even more so with something as important as your health. To put it in layman's terms better yet, simply think about that concept; "would I (insert name here) quit my job if so & so did it? Would you jump off the proverbial cliff if your friends did it? Hopefully the answer is a resounding no or whatever Kool-Aid you're currently drinking should be put down immediately. Losing weight or changing your life for the better in general is going to take a sacrifice. That sacrifice is you! Your old habits, ways of thinking, even potentially your environment must change in order to support healthy growth and simple human productivity. Without a healthy environment both inside and out your odds of success are greatly decreased. Can you still lose weight regardless of changing anything? No.

 You must change to make long lasting, positive habits stick. The change must come from within to without in order to see your dreams come to life. There is no better feeling than for man and woman to struggle with an ideal & finally see it come to fruition in their natural life. You must make that change inside, if you want to change the outside. You can make that change inside, in order to change the outer world. Ask yourself the following when you consider your current habits & decisions. "Is what I'm doing right now, moving me forward or backward?" I'm not saying you have to live a life of constant work, day in & day out. Balance certainly is key. But what I am saying is sometimes, in order to "capture" the island you must burn the boats.

 Cast off any negative thoughts, lovers, quarrels, habits that weigh you down like a ball & chain & become the man or woman you have imagined yourself to be. Before you begin this journey physically, make a stand that you will put yourself first. In turn, that selfishness later on will help others around you as well. Holistic health begins with introspection & initiative. Be relentless in your endeavors, & ruthless with your discipline. Take no prisoners. Including yourself.

 In the grand scheme of things. We, & only we can truly determine our future. Some may wait for inspiration or catastrophe to happen in order to get moving, & I myself was in that "class" so to speak. But I ask now, why wait for such things to happen? Why wait for the unfortunate end in order to rise anew? Has society coddled us into a false sense of comfort, in a number of ways we willingly fall victim too? Or is it just human nature to force adaptation in times of dire need?

We can ask these questions day by day & come to several different conclusions all on our own. Regardless, one fact remains the same; time is still moving, whether you believe in the construct or vehemently oppose it. Your decisions to make improvements & further your growth are only in your hands. Now, more than ever I believe that to be true. In today's world it is much easier to be independent, & ever moving forward, blazing your own path. But it takes a mountain of courage to separate yourself from the heard & become what you truly desire. During your weight-loss journey or overall growth you will have people that will shun you for your change. Understand that a portion of that is that subconsciously they are now threatened by your change because it will then challenge their belief system & lifestyle. Which is of no offense to them, that is how humans are wired. We are born innately to find comfort in repetition. That's just how it is! But since humans have developed the ability to reason, one must ask themselves "What else can I become?" Then aspire to achieve those goals. Whether the support is there, or not.

 So, I ask you; what or who could you be if you were the very best version of yourself?

Chapter 3 - Complaining, the invisible privilege

Here in the U.S., we have a privilege that none of us talk about, but all of us are privy too. That privilege is complaining! The ability to sit around & sulk is not a new notion. Humans have been sitting around for years. Now here's the kicker; procrastination (complaints distant cousin) can be a good thing. Now, don't run to the hills with that one. Complaining & doing nothing about your situation can destroy your dreams, especially if you allow the pressure to take over. It happens. But procrastination with "massive action" can have some results. This example is most prevalent in crash dieting. Even though yes in some instance's procrastination can be a good thing however, in most cases whereas consistent action is required, the idea of "putting it off" spells doom for just about anyone who tries. But, how can we use procrastination to our advantage? We'll touch upon it briefly here but go in depth later on. For this procrastination example, let's take a look at one of music's most polarizing individuals in the 17th century, Mozart. Yes, Mozart.

Wolfgang Amadeus Mozart was born on January 27th, 1756 in the city capital, Salzburg in Austria. Now before he became the Justin Bieber of his time, he already showed signs of "prodigious" behavior within his musical abilities in his earliest childhood. I was picking my nose in the backyard playing tag with my friends meanwhile at the same age, Wolfgang over here has already transcendent to star status speculation. Life comes at you fast. Already well versed in violin & keyboard he started composing for European Royalty at the age of five years old. The pieces he wrote, "K 1 -5 "in his earlier years were recorded by his father, Leopold Mozart in the Nannerl Notenbuch.

Mozart went on tour to perform within the European Royalty enclave in the Child Prodigy Program. Playing a piece in the courthouse in front of the Prince Maximilian III of Bavaria in Munich, circa 1762, the childhood classical genius showed signs of stardom very early on. So much so his father eventually stopped playing altogether in order to further teach young Mozart.

Mozart's musical genius shines through in his greatest piece created, the composition of Don Giovanni's Overture. The best part of this story is that this creative masterpiece was written the *night before.* Yes, the night before. Here's the story; The date is October 28th, 1787 the night before Don Giovanni's premiere. He had gone out with his friends for drinks the night before the show & while out having fun having, his friend mentioned that he hasn't written the overture for the Opera yet.

Back in school I dreaded writing assignments & waited until the very last minute to get them done. I'm no Mozart, but maybe I was onto something? The young genius went home & immediately got to work on his now known masterpiece. Maybe it was the alcohol in his system, or his wife telling him stories as he was working, either way he created one of the most amazing pieces known to man. In a single night might I add. If that doesn't inspire you to sit around & do nothing, I don't know what will. That is total satire by the way. Mozart & Co didn't even have time to rehearse the piece, they simply assembled & pulled it off without a hitch. Truly one of the most clutch moments in all of history, & certainly to Mozart's career as he received a standing ovation thus catapulting him further into the fame, fray & musical stratosphere of that time.

How does this apply to fitness? It absolutely doesn't. The idea of putting off fitness for a long time is a far cry of what actually needs to be done. Health isn't something that can be put off into your later years. Sacrificing your younger years for the sake of a slew of beers after a hard day's work surely does not pay off like having a functional liver at 55. I don't mean to bash if it sounds like I am, but in issues regarding health I firmly believe they need to be communicated as transparent as possible. The goal is to change the root of the problem, not the "stem" so to speak. If we constantly put band-aids on things we can never get rid of the issue in its entirety. This is why fad diets don't work either. They simply fix the issue at hand. For example; going on a diet for 4 weeks to lose 5 pounds solves the issue of losing five pounds. However, it doesn't solve the unhealthy relationship one may have with food. Yes, it is possible to have a relationship with food & not just the edible pens you use in the bedroom with your partner. Lastly, complaining which we all fall victim to does nothing at all. At this point you can see my position on how I feel about doing nothing in the face of opposition.

But I do have a reasoning for this. When I was getting out of high-school I was still slightly overweight but at this point had lost enough to have some muscle tone on my body. When my brother passed away (Didier) it had put me in a state of victimhood. A dark place where I wouldn't talk to anyone, hangout, or be around. My brother's room was right next to mine, 5 feet apart & he had left the door open. So, in a way I sort of sat there, waiting for him to come through the door. Unfortunately, I began to realize the truth that my brother was truly gone & not coming back. In order to cope, I began eating more junk food, playing more video games, & barely went to the gym. I had ballooned again, feeling worse mentally opposed to physically. Although my body wasn't too far off either.

One day I looked in the mirror. I had just graduated but didn't go to college, had no money, & had no job. No sort of direction. I felt lost & I found myself blaming life for inherently cursing me & my family. "Why did my brother have to die?" "Why did it have to end like this?" Or the one I tried to solve for a really long time was, "Why not me instead?" That night I wanted to go with my brother, but he wanted me to stay home. For years I wanted to go back in time & change the circumstances. Maybe if I was there things would be different. I rationalize that anyone would feel that way during a time of crisis & thus it's ok to loath & have self-pity, these are grim situations indeed because they are all subjective to the individual at that time. But I can tell you why that's not okay. Simply because life still goes on. In the grand scheme of things, you still have to pick up the pieces & move on. It's a harsh reality but a reality nonetheless, at some point you have to ask yourself if you're willing to either quit or get up despite the odds & face your fears, fighting for a better future.

Hating the reflection in the mirror I thought to myself that day about what I wanted my life to be, how I wanted to do it & exactly what I want to do. I made a decision that day to at least try to turn my life around. I started small, no major commitments, I knew I couldn't do that realistically. But, one day turned into three & three into five, I then found myself losing the weight I had gained again & lost more. Proud of my progress & motivated to try life again I wrestled through those months to come back to life. Fitness was my key to my second chance & I really tried at that time to become more that I was at the moment. Little did I know I was setting myself up for what was the greatest decision I have ever made.

 When I became a trainer, it was months after my brother passed away. I made my decision to help others along the way by becoming a Personal Trainer & helping other with the knowledge I obtained from not only my experience, but from what my brother had taught me along the way. Lessons & moment's I can never forget. Each one inspiring the steps I took to come out of the darkness that was my own sadness. Action isn't a cure all, but it can be a means to get out of the quicksand that is a catastrophe in one's life. We all have inner, innate desires that we all strive for but unless we put in the work to obtain them, not quit when it gets tough & see it through to its completion, they will forever simply remain dreams. Figments in your imagination, with infinite potential, living & dying in your head.

 That decision I made to be a coach was a decade ago, & I am very happy that I did. There were some very tough challenges on the road to becoming & being a coach but a journey I decided to take on for myself in dedication to someone else that made my decision firm. We all need a reason why we're doing something. Oftentimes the very things we complain about are the opportunities we can take to change our lives. This is how inventions are born. There is a problem, we create the solution. In my opinion, society needs a shift in perspective about issues. I believe if we can reframe them into challenges or growth opportunities, we find that not only were we capable of overcoming but also becoming impactful & influential along the way. It's easy to see everything as doom & gloom, but what if for a moment we saw these things as challenges? I think these are the catalysts that catapult us to our higher & best self. Fitness may seem like a daunting challenge, but a great way to reframe it in my opinion is "How can I take this time to create the body I want, within the realms of what I genetically have available to me right now?" In other words. "How can I take this opportunity to create a brand new, bangin' body?"

This isn't the time to be PC & now declare fitness isn't completely about looking good. You're right. But also, wrong. When you look in the mirror & appreciate what you look like because you've worked for it, that does wonders for your mental health. Granted you need balance in all things however to appreciate & take care of your body is no crime. If part of your goal is to ultimately look better. Make that your goal! Be aware to not compare yourself to anyone & monitor your progress Wishlist being appreciative of what you worked for. When you can envision a better future for yourself no matter in what sector of your life, you are then called to action. However, the key to making this work is to not look down upon those who do not physically resemble a God or Goddess much like you will in the near future. We're all the same! From stout body to shriveled raisin it is the character of man or woman that defines him or her.

From a metaphysical standpoint, the desires you have, deep within you & uninfluenced by society are spirit speaking to you, in your own voice directly. This is the motivation you get to start on whatever endeavor you have. We only complain when we believe that we truly have no other option because we cannot see beyond our current reality. This is where your imagination has to take place. Buildings aren't simply dropped out of the sky. Someone had to think of the design before beginning to build the building that hundreds will soon call work, school, or home. Humans & the human mind are capable of amazing things, but we simply don't give our imaginations enough credit. As we get older, we get told to stop imagining, why? Imagination is the foundation of human growth in all areas. Without the capacity to see beyond you are limited to the options before you. Whether they are abundant, or scarce. If you see yourself as you are & only as you are you will only be what you are. If you can see beyond what you are, there is hope that it can invoke you to take action.

The sands of time wait for no man or woman, whether he be rich or poor. Healthy or sickly. Death comes for each of us at some point. What we do at that time is greatly determined by our influences but ultimately crafted by our own actions. We can blame our parents, society, the government, or whoever else may seemingly fit the bill. Ultimately however, the shoe is custom made for us, & us only. May you not be consumed by your troubles, but brave enough to extinguish the flames when necessary. When it is all said & done, we alone can move through our obstacle, even if that means doing it with anxiety or fear. There is never any better moment than now & putting off any actions that can propel you or complaining about situations you can control will never move you forward. The time for action is now.

Chapter 4 - Sugar Daddy? Yes. Sugar in your diet? No.

It is at this point I would like to state that guys can be sugar babies too. I just needed an entertaining title, so you'd be moderately interested in the world that is nutrition. Before I jump down this proverbial rabbit hole, I would like to mention that at the time of me writing this book I am a certified coach, but not a certified nutritionist or licensed dietitian. That said, the empirical data I will be sharing with you in an effort you can come to your own conclusion are that of my own experience, as well as reliable scientific resources, & I doubly encourage you to do your own research. However, please be advised that if you use this information, whether here or for the remainder of this book, whether that be information in regard to mental, physical, or nutritional health that you not only come to your own conclusion, but also adhere to this information at your own discretion. I guess that's the professional way of saying, "If you break something, don't sue me." With that said, let's continue.

Humans have been eating since forever. Seriously. Since we were simple biomes, crawling along the ocean bottom eating parasites. When we evolved to larger, shit flinging primates we were still occupied on obtaining as much resources for one concept; eating. Sometimes when I'm eating, I ask myself "why?". Not, "why am I eating this bacon burger?" But why am I; a living seemingly self-sustaining organism eating outside matter & not relying on myself to produce the sustenance I need, like plants (kind of) do? This cannabis – munchies driven inquiry does have some merit. Humans have been eating a wide variety (including ourselves, literally) of things for eons, but it doesn't seem like there is an end all be all answer. To discover why, let's think of two things a) eating as a function & b) why eating doesn't necessarily have a finite answer. Lastly, we'll review a diet strategy that includes a form of procrastination, & how we can actually apply that to our fitness goals. Let's start with the topic "a" first.

What is eating as a function? Or better yet, what happens to the body when we eat, & why do we need to fuel our respective bodies? These answers look obvious, but not really! Often the simplest of ideas are an amalgamation of multiple concepts functioning as one. The digestive process is a tricky one, & nonetheless considerably out of my scope. However, I can point out the obvious reason why we eat (as if no one knows) for nutrients of course! The sole purpose of that bacon burger outside of it being absolutely delicious is that my body needs the nutrients provided within what I'm eating. So that's not the issue. Our battle of the bulge is more of the quality & quantity of food rather the idea of eating in itself. Although, one can mention that eating in excess is obviously harmful to the body. So, what diets work & what diets don't? Let's take a look at the very famous "Paleo Diet".

The Paleo diet derives from the basic principles of its main influence, cavemen. Cavemen were hunters - gatherers. Meaning they only hunted what they needed that day & garnered the fruits & vegetables as they moved about during the Paleolithic Era. Hence the fad's name "The Paleolithic Diet". They mainly ate lean meats, fish, fruits & vegetables during that time. The premise of the new PLD is that of a similar concept, "Eat what you were designed to." Which makes sense. Studies show that cavemen were much healthier in comparison to the modern-day man. However, there are also as many counter claims, questioning the lifespan of "The Caveman" which I think is a misnomer. My "theory" here on the lifespan of said cavemen would be that considering the animal species of that time & the nature of moving about; the lifespan of The Caveman would be relatively short. But that's neither here, nor there.

The argument that this is the way to eat for everyone is an extensive one, however I'd like to counter that with the thought that is it possible not one single way works for everyone when it comes to nutrition? From what I've read hunters - gatherers ate what was available to them. They weren't necessarily keen on what exactly to eat, they just knew they had to eat otherwise they would die. That leads me to come to two things; the foods they ate were more than likely seasonal, depending on their geo location. The second being that, depending on their location, they were eating things that were available to them in their respective area as well. Which would mean they have to vary from location to location.

So how can we say that this one diet in particular is a proven way to eat? This is why I don't necessarily champion one diet strategy. I simply do what works best for me by doing research. On myself. Which is relatively easy to do? Eat something, record the effects of it. How do you feel? Sluggish? Energetic? Of course, there is more to it than that. But nutrition in my opinion does not have to be complicated. Nowadays we shame people for eating meat or cheese, joke on people for only eating vegetables for what? It's not as serious as the words here make it in hindsight, but arguments over this is a real thing, happening in nearly every home in America. Millennials shame Boomers over brisket. Boomers shame Millennials over Kombucha. The battle never ends.

So, what is the right diet? I cannot make that decision for you, nor is that what this book is designed to do. The goal is to put you in the driver's seat & liberate yourself from the shame you feel when you "mess up" your "diet". This leads me to context "b" nutrition is not a one-way street. Here's how it works in regard to what really matters, macro nutrients & caloric intake.

Here's how it works; your calories are a make-up of what is known as macro & micronutrients. For example, if you have a meal that is 1000 calories (goddamn bacon burger) a breakdown of that number would be a percentage of "macronutrients" like fat, carbohydrates, protein. They also consist of "micronutrients" like essential vitamins & minerals. All of these play a role in your body's ability to function at its highest capacity. After all, although it is nice to sit at the dinner table with your loved ones over dinner, food is fuel for the body at the end of it all. Therefore, without being a "nutrition - Nazi" one should take a look into what they are eating on a daily basis, too ensure they are getting the right nutrition that works for them. An obvious general advisory step in foods to avoid eating would certainly be avoid eating fast foods on a consistent basis as they are high in calories. But what about the other micronutrient no one mentions you should consider limiting & or eliminating from your diet? That would be sugar.

I cannot say do not consume sugar, but I can say consider the amount your intake on a daily basis. I love fried Oreos as much as anyone, but it doesn't take a lot of them to put me over the mark of what I consider comfortable for myself. Limiting sugar has a lot of benefits but I cannot suggest quitting cold turkey. However, I do believe I can say the following, based on the research I've done.

Sugar with its tasteful pro's, has a litany of con's as well. Enough cons to make you want to stop eating sugar, which is why I don't have to drive a hard campaign against it. The unfortunate part is how addictive it really is & how pervasive it is in our current foods today. You can find sugar in anything from a McDonald's salad, to tomato sauce. Italian grandmas everywhere would be gravely disappointed if they knew of this. Sugar offers literally nothing but sweetness. Literally. It has zero nutritional value. It is nothing more than a sweet carb that spikes your blood sugar. Your blood sugar & weight loss are closely linked as the ability to burn reserved fat aka your "love handles" rely on a relatively low blood sugar level (in the healthy range).

Sugar does the opposite of that. It spikes your blood sugar levels higher than Ike & Tina on a Friday night. Besides ruining your blood sugar levels, it can increase hunger by increasing the ghrelin in your body which is the hormone that promotes the eating "signals" you get when you're hungry. Side note: Hydration & Hunger signals are the same, so oftentimes you may be dehydrated as opposed to actually hungry. Consider your water intake, generally half your body weight in oz will be sufficient to keep you hydrated. Example I weigh 168lbs, so I try to drink 84oz of water. It helps keep track as non-neurotically as possible using a fitness, or nutritional app. Lastly, overconsumption of sugar can come with a host of medical issues as well as mental health complications. Sugar doesn't have to be the demon ruining your life, anything in moderation can be fine as long as you keep it within those parameters. The problem comes from overconsumption & the onset addiction you get from overeating sugar.

So, what is optimal when it comes to dieting? Again, I cannot come to that conclusion for you, but we can go over the fundamentals. I believe if you have the fundamentals down in any subject you can always customize it & make it your own when you are versed in the subject. The fundamentals for nutrition are similar in that regard. Remember, we need food as fuel primarily therefore we need a good number of macronutrients such as fats, protein, & carbohydrates. Don't forget the micronutrients as well. These would be your vitamins & minerals. One might be asking at this point, "what foods provide these nutrients?" Two things I would say to that would be, do the research! This is the time where you can now learn how to eat differently without the confusion. By merit of quality, we can determine that fast food is not the food that should be put on that list.

Google has been the greatest tool to date, for modern man. A search for 'healthy foods list' or 'natural foods' would show a whole array of quality foods you can pick that have the nutrients the human body needs to function properly. I also decided to not include a list because there is also a litany of foods I don't know as well. This is the time for all of us to explore & put together something that works for us as individuals. This is an ever-evolving thing! Your taste will change over time so one cannot assume they will continue to eat off of a list for their entire life. Make it a lifestyle & make healthy eating yours! I can only provide resources & experience that has helped me.

Speaking of things that have helped me, fasting was one of the eating choices I've made that work for me. I started fasting when I was in my early 20's. I was experimenting with dieting strategies & still eating three meals a day. I ate as healthy as what I thought at the time possible, but the weight did not come off at the rate I would like. This is around the time I started making a comeback to the gym but wasn't totally focused on nutritional value. When I got a job at GNC, I'd have work in the morning. So, because I was never the type to wake up early, I'd also wake up and have to rush for work because I relied on public transportation. So, I often skipped breakfast as a result of that. When I noticed the weight coming off, I credited my gym efforts, but I did make note that it could possibly be to me not eating as normal as I would. This sparked my curiosity on the idea of fasting, & till this day (my late 20's) it has become more of a lifestyle.

Remember that whole bit on procrastination & applying it to fitness? Fasting is it. Fasting has a whole host of benefits, & with recent information being published it's easy to see why it's becoming a trend among fitness enthusiasts everywhere. The idea of "putting off" your nutrition applies perfectly in this regard. Fasting or IF (Intermittent Fasting) allows the digestive system to "clean" itself in regard to waste products & metabolize the stored fat cells that you have in your body. This method of eating is not suitable for those with medical conditions, including but not limited to diabetes. Also, if you're new to the idea of it, I would not recommend diving in headfirst.

My eating window is one massive meal a day, with a 18-24 hour fasting window shortly after that. Your eating window does not have to be as long. If you skip dinner at 7pm (meaning you stop eating at 6pm) go to bed on an empty stomach & eat breakfast at 7am, that's already 13hrs without trying. I used to count calories & weigh out my food but not anymore. Remember the idea is to make things less complicated, & when you break your fast you want to eat quality, natural foods.

I also changed what I was looking for in sound nutrition. I focused on eliminating the sugar, more protein, moderate carbs, fiber & a healthy amount of fats (of course I'm addicted to "guac"). As of recently I also eliminated the bacon burgers from my life & eat a more plant-based diet with a kink for seafood on occasion. When people ask why I switch I always make it clear it's not for ethical reasons, but someone said something to me so casual to me it shifted my perspective. "The meat you eat doesn't eat meat; it eats plants. The same plants you eat."

With that thought I was inspired to change, & after watching a video of little chicks being shuffled into a grinder whilst chirping, I made a firm decision to move away from all chicken-based products, However I'm not hung up on the idea. No matter how noble not eating meat is for the sake of animal lives, and I myself being predominately "plant based, I still believe dieting should inherently be flexible & a personal choice. One cannot concretely conclude someone's proper nutritional setup outside of being a doctor assigned to said patient, or a nutrition specialist hired by said client. As humans we have lived all over this beautiful world eating a wide array of foods, dictated by what was available to them & I for one will never turn down a well cooked, rare T-bone steak when I'm traveling through the south. Crucify me if you will but at least honor my transparency. For example, look at the Potato Famine in Ireland. The survivors ate a diet that consisted of "corn, oats, potato, wheat & milk stuffs".

Should we be toting that as the new end all be all of nutrition? Of course not! My point here is diets should be malleable to the user. Consider what works for you in regard to calorie intake, & nutritional value, whether that be brisket, or beans. Or both, those two go very well together.

In conclusion, diets or the idea itself should be a lifestyle. The approach of doing this for a certain amount of time & the ongoing back to your old ways is a bad idea & leads to less than desirable results. We have a fear of exploring the unknown, shunning others for doing it or us ourselves stopping for fear of being criticized by our peers. Society does a great job of dictating our desires without us even knowing. How many times have you "cheated" on your lifestyle simply because it was easier to deal with as opposed to listening to your friends gripe & hitting you with "You only have one life just eat the damn cake." To be fair, they have a point. Eat the damn cake.

However, the reality is somewhere along that week we already abandoned our new lifestyle for that leftover cheesecake from your nieces christening. Here you are, destroying it at 3am in the morning. Then the next day you rationalize your previous behavior with a run. Only to follow that up with an iced latte before you head into the office. Friday then comes around & here you are with your friends, thinking your head about the previous infractions you committed.

 These little cheat moments we have in our diet are always hidden setbacks. Yes, did you earn that cheesecake after 3 days of being "good"? Sure. But consider you have a life & odds are that you will be dining with your friends at some point later in the week. What if you thought of calories like a savings bank? Work hard all week & have a balanced but fun time on the weekend? There's no need for the pressure or self-shame you may feel if you stay the course during the week, when it absolutely counts. You owe it to yourself to keep that promise. People have the propensity to let us down, even if they don't mean it. Why do it to ourselves? Work hard, save your "calorie dollars" for the weekend & get a well-deserved break. Balance your fasting with sound nutrition that works for YOU based on the research YOU or the person you hired (or doctor) prescribes. Remember that no one can experience your body (in this context) & ultimately you or the person you hired has to do the research & come to a decision that works for you. Eat right, keep your promise to yourself & eat the damn cake.

 The topic of nutrition is a boring one (at least to me), however I hope the topics we had set out to discover in this chapter were clearly communicated to you in a way that was entertaining, informative & motivates you to start your own nutritional research, paired with your own experience. Going forward we will talk about things more within my scope by way of functional fitness. Let's get into the "meat & potatoes" of the next chapter. Pun fully intended.

Chapter 5 - Attack on Titan

Personally, I hate the fitness industry. Or at the very least I hate what it's become. In a world now full of social media (".Fits" of Instagram. I am one myself.) shock jocks, voicing bro science all in the name of likes, fit chicks who get procedures done & rep "detox" teas, it's easy to understand why there is so much misinformation & confusion within the fitness world. I think for the exception of some individuals & brands within the "game" truly care about the consumer of their information or product. Capitalism is a great tool, but it can ruin those with even the best intentions. Also, this is not to virtue signal in any way shape or form. I am totally in this for the money as well as impact. I, much like you have expenses! That is not my focal point. It is merely a byproduct I am happily conscious & privy too.

We as a society can create something of value & still be able to receive some form of acknowledgment for it but it has to benefit the consumer as well! This is a two-way street, & I believe with the information I provide within this book "paves the road" itself so to speak. My goal is to provide clear concise information that is replicable for you, the reader. If I sold you a program, you'd always be in a position of "helpless consumerism" however if I can teach you how to coach yourself, I am confident you will be able to make progress on your own, & when the time comes for a coach, you will have some no how as to what to look for in a good trainer. Remember your body is your biggest investment!

So, where to from here? In this chapter I'll be discussing some methods you can apply to your workout program in regard to workout creation & optimization. We'll learn about what "Quad Sets" are & how we can put exercises in order to fit the program set up. We'll talk planes of motion & what they mean in relation to your program. We'll talk about warmups, & cool downs as well. This is the point where I would suggest taking notes if not already, & attempt to put together a program as well. As a final note I'd like to advise that with all exercises you decide to put into your program, you take on the risk & also assume you know the extent of your limitations. Because this is a book & I am not literally present with you at the moment, I can only create structure for you, but you have to take on the risk & responsibility of performing the exercises you chose in accordance to these methodologies. Now if I didn't scare you away, let's begin!

Okay, planes of motion. What are they & why do you need to know? The human body is capable of some truly remarkable things. That is one of the things that first drew me into fitness post the passing of my brother. Wanting the changes made me start, seeing the changes kept me going. Outside of the body's ability to shift physiologically, from an anatomical standpoint we shine here as well. Ranges of motion delegate what the body can do in its relation to the space and objects surrounding or possibly equipped at the time. In addition to that, various joints within the body have what I like to call single degree functions. For example, using your shoulder, you can rotate the arm so that the bone positioned on the inside of the forearm (ulnar) is now externally exposed. This would make the shoulder joint a "global joint".

However, a motion like a bicep curl is different. You can only hinge the elbow joint to & away from the body. You cannot rotate the ulnar so that it faces externally from the body like the shoulder & please do not try. With the limited range of motion in the elbow joint, this would be called a "local joint". The same joint systems can be found in the hips, wrists, knees, ankles. All of these joint patterns make up human movement as a whole from a skeletal perspective. Muscle also plays a role in motion and motor control has more to do with the core, hips, & glutes which will be discussed later on within this chapter.

There are major planes of motion that the body as a whole performs day in & day out. The biggest one of them being rotation, which I would consider is often left out of most workout programs, or inefficiently executed, doing more damage to the lumber (lower portion of the spine.) instead of chiseling out the sought after "Adonis Belt" V - taper. The official term for the plane of motion is called The Transverse plane. This plane of motion is responsible for the rotation of the body, as stated above. The main muscle that uses the rotation primarily is the core. Did you know walking is a transverse plane of motion? This is debatable actually. Science by definition tells us that the act of walking is a forward motion by nature, unless you strut like a penguin. However, I'd argue that the muscles responsible for the body's forward movement through space is the core! Also, the glutes as well as they provide more support for balance when walking.

Another main reason why rotations are good for the body are the obliques & their responsibility in relation to movement. The core is made up of multiple muscles, such as the internal/external obliques located on the sides of the torso, transverse abdominis which is the external & lateral portion of the torso, & finally the rectus abdominis which is also external, but runs vertically. The RA makes up your "washboard" abs, internal - external obliques are buried under your love handles, & your transverse abdominis keeps it all together like a belt in the front & defines your "v-line." Note that all these muscles are found in both sexes although they may not be held to such high priority in regard to the person creating & or using the program.

From my years of being a coach, including my own training in my early years both personal & professional I've always either had slight back pain, or my clients had back pain. From countless trial & error, I've come to learn that the core (with many "sub" muscles included) is responsible for both proper posture & back pain. The better you can develop your core & strengthen those muscles through stabilization (remember the core is also a proponent of proper balance.) the better your back will feel & your posture will also improve. So, in short, your back pain is due to a tight back, & weak core.

Now in hindsight this sounds like a no brainer, & this is merely an overview of these functions, you would think you can find this information easily. Even as coaches we often fall prey to misinformation. A true testament is something working on you first, & then can it only be applied to someone else. With this logic, one can see how these exercises can be left out if not checked for, professional or otherwise. Hopefully with this book it can encourage you to do some research on exercises that work for you whether you have back pain or not. Chiseled cores aren't just for looks; they also have some function! Consider a rotation exercise like a standing or kneeling chop for your program. In regard to stabilization, consider something like a plank.

Stabilization exercises are often "timed" exercises so there isn't necessarily a reason to add a rep scheme to a plank. You're better off timing it, for example 30 - 45 seconds. There are various stabilization & strengthening exercises that not only make them look good but perform better. Consider doing some trial & error to determine which feels right for you & YOUR body.

The next plane of motion we have is called The Frontal Plane. By definition, it is responsible for splitting the movement of the body into front & back halves. Typically, the movements associated with this plane of motion would include things such as going up & down, or side to side. Think movements like Back Squat, Pull-up, & Shoulder Press. All of these movements move in an up & down pattern. Depending on your orientation in relation to space, the glute bridge would be another example of this plane of motion.

The glute bridge should be a staple in your exercise program because it has multiple functions depending on how you perform the movement. The muscle primarily activated in this are the glutes, which are actually split into three. We have the "Gluteus" Maximus, Glute Med, & Glute Minimus. They are positioned exactly how they sound but for a grand overview we have the Max positioned at the top portion of the butt, the Med which covers the middle portion, & the Minimus which is located towards the bottom end of the glutes, towards the hamstring area. These muscles serve various functions but the main one I am inferring to is its ability to help stabilize the body & alleviate lower back pain by strengthening the glutes entirely.

Other movement concepts within this plane involve the back squat which is often associated with the main "lifts" you'd want to incorporate into your program as well. These main lifts are the Deadlift, Back Squat, Bench Press (or pushup), Pullup, & for arguments sake I would say the side lunge with just about anything you can do it with. Weight or otherwise. Primarily this is also a movement pattern not always used during program creation. These "lifts" include some of the major muscle groups in the body such as the Pecs (chest), Lats (back), Quads (front portion of the thigh) & the Glutes (...butt). Note that there are many smaller muscles in conjunction with the muscles mentioned previously, this is a great time to begin to fill your own knowledge bank with more terms associated. Consider adding these movements to your workout program, regardless of goal.

 Strength is an important aspect of any workout program. Whether you're looking to "get calendar" ready or want to finally beat up your older siblings after 20 plus years of sibling rivalry, you need to add these movements into your program for they are the foundation of movement in its entirety. Besides, who doesn't like to bust out 50 pushups during your cousin graduation BBQ? I know I do. Strength also helps with maintaining bone density as you age. Gravity has a funny way of shrinking us as we get older without really realizing, & when your bones are weak, they are more susceptible to breaking & other conditions. Stop getting outlifted by grandmas (no hate!) & add some strength to your program. Your muscles, & bones will thank you.

 The last plane of motion to cover is the Sagittal Plane. This plane of motion splits the body into left & right, & the movements associated with it are often moving forward & back. More dynamic in nature. Think running, walking, back extensions & even bicep curls. The back plays a role in this movement function in relation to the muscle groups. Essentially the back is mainly for pulling, not inherently lifting although your lower back plays a role in that as well. The Latissimus Dorsi or "lats" as the bros call it are one of the largest muscle groups in the body. This muscle takes on the role of pulling things to you, pulling yourself upwards, & not to mention further supporting your torso.

 Back exercises are primarily important because of the postural benefits they provide, beyond the strength aspect. A well-defined back not only looks good to the voyeurs, but it also provides the strength necessary to help you carry your best friend's couch up to his new apartment, conveniently located on the 8th floor...with no elevator. The lats lock into the body like a suture when you're carrying something or performing a pulling movement. Oftentimes clients may note that they cannot feel the lats working, regardless of its size in relation to the body.

 The key here is to create a mind muscle connection to feel the muscle & mind in order to activate the muscle. It should be no surprise to any of us to find out the body is controlled by the brain. The brain is made of various microscopic matter but also neurons. Neurons run signals throughout the Nervous System stimulating every movement & impulse in the body, so it would be imperative to work on mind muscle development. Think about when you're driving home from work. Sometimes you "blank", not consciously navigating the road & still make it home? Why? Neural pathways embedded in the brain help develop a pattern or "sequence" giving the brain directions without you consciously being aware. This is like Tesla's autopilot function, only a little more dangerous but a lot cheaper.

So, we know neurons send messages throughout the body like a superhighway, & we often do this unconsciously. How do we not only use this for fitness but also do this consciously, & willingly? A couple methods have shown how this could be done. Let's consider flexing the muscles in between sets for example. You don't have to be Arnold to flex in the gym, in fact you may not even need a mirror at all, although it helps for posing & in my opinion, can't hurt!

After your performed set, flex the muscle you just used for the same amount of reps, then take a break. The idea is to further stimulate the muscles, getting the neurons to fire off within the fibers causing your brain to remember to activate that muscle when the contraction is occurring. You may not notice at first but over time you will be able to contract the muscle easier, making it easier to target specifically & fatigue it much faster. A great all-around exercise that not only strengthens the Lats, trains the Sagittal Plane & strengthens the core would be the farmers carry. The weights don't have to be dramatically heavy, just ensure proper distance between your start & finish. Note that you should always check your ego at the door & test all weight prior to lifting it.

Ah yes, the ego. The thing that makes you send those late-night drunk texts at 2am. "Are you up?" you send, staggeringly yet eagerly making your way to your taxi. We humans have evolved with the ability to reason. A blessing & a curse. The ego cuts corners for the sake of comfort, barters your future aspirations for temporary pleasures & can buy you a one-way ticket to "Snap City" if you're not careful checking your weight. You can get away with some "ugly" lifts if the movement allows it. In other words, if you're doing an exercise such as a Burpee for instance, we can allow *some* degree of "form manipulation" in regard to how the exercise is to be properly performed. A kettlebell swing? Not so much. A heavy weight being moving dynamically can spell doom for your lower back if you're not accustomed to the weight itself, let alone if you have never done the movement.

What is the best strategy in this case? Consider progressive overloads. Each week as you progress through your program, simply add 5lbs to the weight of the exercise. Example say you were to perform a bench press at 100lbs for about 10 repetitions last week. This week add 5lbs bringing your weight to 105lbs. The chances of you hitting the 10-rep mark are still high, but the added weight provides the weight necessary in order to stress the fibers, promoting growth & forcing adaptation. In this case, the idea of jumping 10lbs plus per week would be a gross exaggeration of what the human body was capable of in relation to a new "environment". Muscles were made to aid the human in movement so in this regard & my professional opinion. Progress overloads provide the body the means to get stronger & minimizes the risk of injury as well. Fitness is a long journey, & you only get one fresh set of joints before having to see the doctor for new, mechanical ones. Consider putting that off for as long as possible.

When I was growing up, my mom gave me an allowance, when she could. She taught to save "whatever I could" for rainy days. Naturally I did not adhere to this advice at first. But as we all know, life comes at you full circle. Now when I think back to every dollar I've ever made; a moment of regret always comes over me. If I had listened to my mother at a young age, through the power of compound interest (or even just saving money in a piggy bank) I would have a lot more to my name that I do now. The notion also implies strength training & weight loss. Every exercise you do should have some variation of progression that works for you. Of course, we want basic safety precautions to ensure longevity, but some areas need to be stressed specifically to ensure growth. If you simply add 5lbs to your program over 12 weeks, how much stronger & or leaner could you be?

With a lot of my older clients that are new to exercise, my strategy for adding variations & stressors are within the floor exercise category. When a newer client initially starts a workout program, the idea is to work from the floor up. This is something I would recommend you add into your program progression. You start from the floor, lying on your back to a full kneeling position. As you get stronger you progress these movements from full kneeling to a half kneeling position & finally on your feet. The reason for this is although many of the other exercises for the remainder of the workout may be on the feet, we can take advantage of strengthening the muscles through these phases with body weight or minimally resisted exercises, later on letting them loose on more robust movements.

The overall takeaway here in this chapter is that you should consider all planes of motion & the weight you use when creating your new workout program. Strength plays a vital role in weight loss & it's important for me to mention also that weightlifting does not turn you into a body builder overnight. The men & women that are within that "bracket" to say have spent decades working out & using extra credit substances in order to achieve the look necessary for these competitions. Unless those are your goals, the chances of this happening to you are small. In fact, what will actually happen is you raise your metabolic rate, making your body burn calories at rest easier because it has more muscle density it has to supply energy for. So ideally, the stronger you get the easier your body melts fat without doing anything. That's not a magic pill by any means, but the idea that your body is more efficient through training should be enticing to anyone looking to drop a couple pounds or make a major lifestyle change.

Lastly, remember Rome wasn't built in a day. Seriously. Rome took 1,009,491 days to build Rome. Seriously! That is also if you consider its "sacking" over time & the date at which the city was founded, April 21st 753 BCE. With that said, you will also need to develop two key skills in order to ensure your success. Those would be consistency, & patience. What is consistency? Simply put the idea to do something over & over again, day in, day out. I would also say regardless of circumstance as well, although at times it is necessary to take a break. However, when you are consistent, you are simply building on the day before, improving your chances of making your goal tangible & further along the road to success. Consistency is only half of the equation, but a rather important one at that.

 What is patience? Patience is the ability to accept or tolerate delay, trouble or suffering without getting angry or upset. This is a game changer in the world of fitness, stocks, or just about anything that actually matters in life. Strip away the modern era of its instant gratification & watch as the world descends into chaos. We now are used to a lot of processed material that comes in all forms. Junk Tv, junk political propaganda, & junk food. Even junk supplements. Your results won't be noticeable for about 12 weeks to be completely transparent.

Any trainer worth their salt has no problem being transparent with you, however sometimes that's not the case. Because coaches must also sell training packages, any notion that you're in it for the long haul can sound daunting when you're shelling out thousands. Same applies to your own workout program. On the road you will slip up, you will hit "potholes" & sometimes you will be down on yourself because you yourself haven't seen the major change that you're looking for. I'm telling you, as the man that (for exception for Mr. White himself) went from "Urkel to Jaleel" patience is the virtue that will give you the strength to keep going & consistency is the vehicle that will get you there. Before you know it, you'll be turning heads & breaking (not literally) necks everywhere you go. But more importantly, you'll be proud of yourself that you stuck to something, & made it happen.

Chapter 6 - System Settings

Last chapter we covered the planes of motion & what their primary roles are in the body. Knowing what they are, which muscles move which, & why they are necessary is only half the battle! The next question I had for myself when I was first coming across this information was "Knowing what I know now, how do I put together a program that works for me, but can also be effective for ME?" Remember, fitness is not a one size fits all & to be quite frank, the act of moving essentially burns calories. Those chores you do? Calorie burning. Chasing your kid around to put them to bed? Calorie burning. *Dirty Dancing* in the house alone in your underwear to your favorite track? You guessed it, calories.

So why in this case does the majority of the fitness industry demand that each workout is a mini Navy Seal Crucible? I love hard workouts. What I can be honest & say is I absolutely loathe hard workouts when I was starting out at 13. Now? If my heart isn't pounding out of my chest, I most likely did yoga. However, that was something I grew into, not a sudden jump into something such as CrossFit that so many unfortunately decide to do.

You never have a "new to fitness" client start out with burpees. That's a great way to lose clients & even quicker way to gain the nickname "Sargent" without ever stepping foot in military gear. The reality is we want to ease into the fire. Consider the cruel yet true story about the frog in the pot. If you were to throw a frog in a pot of boiling water, it will definitely jump out. But if you gradually raise the temperature over time, that frog will sit in the pot comfortable without ever realizing it's being prepared to be an appetizer at your local French 5 star.

The same can be said for fitness. The hardest workouts in the world have absolutely no value if you train that style once or do that workout only one time. However, if you can condition your body, every day, one hour, & progress your exercises correctly & towards your goals, you'll be crushing harder workouts in no time. You may not be a David Goggins, but as you continue to work out you will fortify your mind, you will get stronger mentally & you will see the results you're working so hard for provided you stay consistent with what you're doing. Better to start slow & work your way up instead of jumping straight into the deep end.

 Considering the title of the book, I'd imagine you're here primarily to lose weight. Also considering you may be new to fitness; I will be addressing the topic as such. This chapter is about creating your program which entails training frequency, exercise sets & repetitions, progressions, warmups & cool downs. Which may seem like a lot of information to cover but please rest assured once you understand these concepts, they provide a good foundation to build from. To start the topic, we will cover frequency first.

 Frequency. How much is too much, & how much is not enough? First before questioning your frequency, consider how long it takes to recover. If you're new to fitness odds are you will be sore early on. Another reason why I express easing into it. Ever experienced lower back soreness from your first set of heavy deadlifts? That kind of pain can render you practically immobile. If you're new to a movement, consider just working with the bar or something a bit lighter that works for you. Besides onset soreness for most beginners the next type of soreness would be DOMS.

 Delayed Onset Muscle Soreness is a condition that comes from the breakdown of the microscopic tissues within the muscle. When the body experiences a weight it's not used to the muscles will tear in effort to work with the load. However, the muscle repair & come back much stronger in effort to work with the load the next time around. Some more factors that could contribute to your level or soreness include but are not limited to training biological age, chronological age, & hormonal status. Having regular doctor checks up is advisable & ensure that you are physically capable from a medial aspect to undergo exercise as per it does change your heart rate & if you have High or Low blood pressure fast movements or moving vertically is a no go.

 With those things taken into account & your work-life schedule as well, you can create the best schedule that works for you. I usually advise my newer clients to start off with 1 session with me & 2 solo workouts for a total of 3 sessions per week. For you, that may be two workouts alone and one with a coach or completely on your own if you're confident enough to take that on. That in my professional opinion is the perfect foundation to build off of. From there, you can add more workout days to your program including a variation of exercises that are in line with your goals. Rest days are just as important, as the body repairs at rest & during sleep. Nutrition is also the name of the game here as your body will express what you eat outwardly, also having an impact on how the body functions as well. At some point, 3 sessions a week won't be enough for you from a social aspect & fitness as well. I find that if you introduce fitness the right way, where someone is eager to make changes, they are not only likely to stick with it but become a part of the facility's social ecosystem as well. I always thought of personal training as training wheels & at some point the person should be ready to take up the mantle on their own. I think this comes from my brother's passing. It showed me that truly anything can change & eventually what you learn must be put to use, independently.

  So, we know how many days to train, what about the exercises, sets & reps? Here's where most get lost, & that's okay! There is a lot of information out there, & part of our job as individuals is to make informed decisions for ourselves. I can't tell you what exercises to do exactly, But I can give you the structure to build a program with the exercises you pick. Think about it like a buffet, but for your muscles. I believe every person should be able to properly train themselves & have the choice to seek help if they wish. Fitness should never be a have to situation, & I believe when you are more informed about something you are more enthusiastic & more likely to continue on your journey. Let's get started!

  Before anything, I like to start with breath work. There are tons of resources on Google to help you find the type of style that works for you. I like to do it with music & some don't. All good! Deep breathing helps slow down your heart rate, calm your nerves & reframe your state of mine prior to activity. Studies also show that 20 - 30 minutes of deep breathing can actually help burn calories. In regard to deep breathing before a workout it does not have to be that long... people might think you're asleep on the floor at the gym. Consider doing some breathe work for about 5-10 minutes prior to your workout that day. You can do this in the morning when you wake up, but I've personally seen best results from doing it before a workout session. So when you consider your breathe work as a part of your program, you're working out without really trying. Look at you! Off to a good start already.

Next up we have our warmup. Very essential but remember you want to make it dynamic. Dynamic as in moving. For example, a jumping jack or earthworm can be much more beneficial to the elasticity of your muscle fibers & the sheath of tissue that surrounds them (fascia), which is responsible for the stretch reflex. That explains why your body hurts when you try to stretch it. The reflex or fascia in this case is trying to prevent itself from being torn in two. So, in this case, light movement is a little more beneficial to the body. This is not to say stretching doesn't have a place in fitness, this tool is simply more valuable in a Corrective Exercise aspect.

  After the warmup I like to advise my clients to do some form of cardiovascular work in an effort to get the heart rate going. It doesn't have to be stressful, but we are looking to target the fat burning zone of the heart rate specifically. With that in mind, you can find a heart rate calculator online & calculate yours, or better yet you can get a heart rate monitor to monitor your cardiovascular progress in real time. The cardio doesn't have to be running per say. You can do anything you like so long as it gets you in your fat burning cardiovascular range. After the 10 minutes is over it's time to hit the floor and do some glute work & core work.

I like to pair them together because they work in unison, the core stabilizes the body through motion & the leg's both stabilize & transmit the Kinetic Energy from the ground into the body when performing a movement. For this reason, strengthening both the glutes & core help to strengthen the body overall, & improve performance in regard to the body's power output in relation to strength. The exercises don't have to be extremely difficult at first but over time you want to progress the difficulty of all exercises (excluding breathing, warmup, cardio - if you so wish) every two weeks, & the weight associated with the exercise by 5lbs every week as well. In regard to sets, 3 is the optimal amount of times each movement can be performed to achieve failure. Rep range is targeted to fat loss, so it is best to aim for 15 - 20 reps depending on the exercise & make that per side when doing single sided exercises.

Once those movements are done, you are now ready for the real workout. Yes, the real workout. The good news is, this doesn't have to be impossible! What works for you, does just that. Just be sure you're challenging yourself whenever possible through progressions. The exercises should be 4 full body movements you can do for about 15 - 20 reps, whether that be with weight or not. Note that there should be no breaks during these 4 exercises until the last exercise of the first round within the circuit is finished

For example, let's say you have chosen these movements as your four exercises (earthworm, pushup, plank, glute bridge). You will complete each exercise in that order, and only take a break after the completion of all the reps for the fourth exercise.

You will do 3 sets or "rounds" for each exercise. After the round is complete go ahead & take a 60 - 90 second break. People tend to use their phone here at this time, don't. You'll be more likely to lose focus & your heart rate will drop. Not a catastrophe, but leaving that fat burning zone will stop you from doing just that. Besides, this is YOU time. Why give up your precious minutes to be alone, & be at peace masochistic style? You owe it to yourself to take this moment to sweat out, anything!

After the torture comes 1 final round of HiiT. That is short for High Intensity Interval Training. The idea of hiit is to do one movement intensely for a set duration of time. In this case we've already done a full-blown workout, so now we want to just use this as "icing" for our torture cake. For that reason, pick an easy to moderately difficult (depending on your experience) conditioning movement, and perform it at 80-95% intensity for 60 seconds. That's it, very low commitment. Again, this can be any exercise that can do for a certain period of time, & it must be cardiovascular based. The idea is to promote more fat loss after the workout is over. After your cool down however, go ahead & finish off with a cool down. Usually light stretching & or breath work helps re-center the mind, bringing the heart rate back down to normal levels.

Viola! You've created your first workout. Now from here you can do the same workout again for the next 2 sessions, & for the next two weeks. Keep mind that you're adding 5lbs per week & progressing the exercises themselves every 2 weeks on top of that. Take your time with your workout & feel it out. Literally. Take a note of how you feel after everything you do. It doesn't have to be neurotic or obsessive. Taking stock of how you feel in real time consciously is a great way to note what changes to make after the session is over. This way, we increase the chances of success & progress throughout the program. Be sure to log your work, I find this best to be done with a notebook, but with the advent of technology plenty of fitness apps include this feature, or you could use your note pad.

Now you may have read this entire section, created your program but still may feel a little unsure of what to do next in terms of progression. Admitting the research is hefty, something not a lot of people can genuinely commit time to learning thoroughly which is completely understandable!

Which is why Scintilla PT is such a passion project for me. Growing up, I didn't always have the access to a lot of the information that is available now on today's internet, so I had to learn a lot on my own. Which then begs the question, "If I had a hard time with it, how many other people do?" To reiterate my mission statement from the chapters before; My goal is to provide the masses proper, high quality Personal Training to the masses at a price point that doesn't break the bank.

If you've come the "crossroads" of your fitness journey and not sure what route to take next, head to www.scintillapt.com and book your first consultation with us. During the zoom (at the time of writing) we can discuss different strategies you can implement into your own program. Think about me as your fitness tutor!

Of course, if you're also looking for coaching you can still head to the same website and fill out the new client profile form. After taking a look at your profile, we'll get your program set up within 24 hours or less.

After becoming a client, you'll have access to 3 zoom meetings per month with your coach to keep you on track. Not to mention the exclusive app you'll have access to. From there you can view easy to follow video instructions from our virtual coaches to help maximize your gym sessions and get the body you deserve once and for all.

Scintilla PT. Innovation Personified.

Chapter 7 - There is no finish line

There is no finish line. Let me explain. Growth inherently has no end for the exception of one's perception within the body they live in & space they occupy. With said I have a question; Have you ever seen an Oak Tree grow halfway? I never have. Why do we as humans find complacency to be the end goal? In a world where you can be anything you can in this "uni" or even "multiverse" we choose the easy way out most of the time. If we all know we are inherently on the greatest game show known to man, why are we all not playing it at the biggest stakes? Or rather, why not go for the grand prize? Obviously, I cannot shame someone for wanting to live in their own respective bubble. But I think this is wrong, and here's why.

I was watching *David Goggins* on the *Joe Rogan Podcast* & he mentioned something about there being no "finish line" per say. When I heard that I had to think about what he meant, & then what it meant to me. Wondering how I could apply that to my life, I've come to the realization, much like Goggins did, that the simple act of living in itself is a race. As you progress through life you begin to craft what your ideal situation would be & then you act on it. *That is the race*. Progress learn & become more. One achievement does not inherently mean you should stop aspiring to achieve more. In fact, it's time to ramp it up.

Imagine you had the chance to "enhance" your abilities like running, jumping, strength, intelligence etc. Wouldn't you want to essentially "max" out these powers? If life had sliders, wouldn't you turn them all the way up? What I'm trying to get at here is life itself can be viewed as a game, whereas the more you train your "powers" the more abilities you have. If you're stronger you can lift heavier things. Smarter people can understand processes a lot quicker & apply them more efficiently. Creative people can create more immersive art using various outlets & etc. The universe or whatever you call what could be the greater powers at hand, has granted us the capability to max out our abilities given that we are willing to put in the work. So, what are we afraid of?

I think we're afraid of not being either able to maintain our newfound glory or won't be able to measure up to what we see as the ideal life for us. But I think there is a reframing that should be in order. Essentially life is about nothing more than growth & contribution. Our society has a dark underbelly for the love of mediocrity. I don't think the blood is on our hands rather. Think about the last time you had a conversation with someone. Remember the time you mentioned to someone you had a certain aspiration, & you mentioned it in hopes the person would both encourage you & also share a dream of theirs, only to shun you for having higher aspiration than what they could realize at the time? Projecting their fears onto your dreams? That's a downer. Mainly it's a downer not because you finally realize your friend isn't that supportive, but because you realize how pervasive that mindset really is.

The book *Mindset* by Psychologist & Researcher Carol S. Dwek explains this perfectly in full depth, & with robust information. To learn more about these two mindsets in full depth I highly suggest viewing her work. But essentially what she explains is that you live with either two mindsets, fixed or growth. The names give away exactly the two terms meaning but its breakdown is what gives more information. Fixed mindsets believe they cannot change their circumstances regardless of opportunities. When you feel you're unable to generate change, you begin to feel as if you always have to prove yourself, using the same old methods you have tried before thus perpetuating the failure cycle further reinforcing your previous notion.

I remember a short while ago while writing this book I had stopped for about 3 months. During that time, I had lost motivation due to the current life & times (Circa 2020 - The Covid era) & was having an existential crisis, mixed with a little depression every other day like I was back in 2011. Or even in 2018. I had lost what I felt was my purpose & after seeing the current state of what the country was, I had a bleak look on my future as a coach in NYC. As time went on however, things got better. At my lowest I had re-confirmed my decision to never have a fixed mindset & reminded myself to see the silver lining in all things. Happily, to announce this sent shockwaves to the rest of the things I've needed to do in my personal life reminding me that we are truly capable of overcoming things, but it starts with our mind.

A growth mindset is exactly that. Growth. The deeper meaning to it, to me personally is one person that is able to see the opportunities that are around them. Making the best & learning from every situation, even with the things they failed trying. When you have a stock & it tanks, you only lose essentially on paper. In other words, unless you hit 'sell' it's not really a loss because of the stocks ability to bounce bank. This is exactly how the growth mindset works. & I fully agree with it. Your chances of success do increase when you fail, but the defining factor is if you are keen on noting the mistakes that have been made, & your ability to apply the correct knowledge the next time around, when the opportunity strikes.

Einstein said once "insanity is doing the same thing over & over, expecting a different result every time." There is some real merit to what has been said there mainly because throughout society & our own lives we tend to do the same thing over & over again in hopes that things change. Just think back to that super toxic relationship you had sophomore year of college. You stuck around thinking things could change & things would get better but alas, it didn't work. Why? We tend to throw Band-Aids on all things we feel we cannot change. But the essence of life itself is having the ability to see what opportunities are in the change, & "lean into it" as Ralph Waldo Emerson once famously said.

 At the end of the day, who we are & who we want to become are only a matter of time & action. The game show is life, & the grand prize is making all your dreams come to fruition. The clock is ticking, & we're not sure when the plug will be pulled. So why live life thinking we know it all? Why wander through life with an air of arrogance disguised as complacency? We complain about how our lives should be more vibrant, more robust, more alive yet here we are with the ability to make a change, a long lasting one at that, & we do nothing until we feel we absolutely have too?

 This is the plight of the human mind & the human condition. The bane of our species' existence. If you have a fixed mindset you simply live life through a fixed, stubborn ideal which can hinder your progress & overall sense of happiness in life. I don't think life is mainly about being happy, but I can certainly say you're better off being happy as opposed to without, that's for sure. Seeing the world through a "half empty lens" is nostalgic at best, implying your fixed ways mean something to you. But they are also detrimental at worst, considering your inability to change.

 But time, much like your fear is also irrelevant. Let me explain, again. The idea of time has no place in the construct of the universe. It is our ability of being cognizant of the change during the day, that we associate the idea of time too. Without being aware of change taking place in the space you occupy; how would you know what time it is? What we're really measuring here is entropy. What is entropy you say? Well as my friend Samuel L. Jackson once famously put "Hold onto your butts." cause' I'm going to tell you. However, if this information does intrigue you, feel free to do some self-study!

 For starters, entropy is still a mystery to scientists that do research on this topic for their livelihood, so the scope of my knowledge albeit accurate due to research, is only a microcosm of what is known. Entropy can be best described as a measurement of disorder in the Universe. "The Second Law of thermodynamics states that the entropy can never decrease" in other words forever expanding. In this case, one could question if time is linked to entropy & you may be correct. According to Wikipedia "entropy is the only quantity in the physical sciences (apart from certain rare interactions in particle physics) that requires a particular direction for time, sometimes called an arrow of time. As one goes "forward" in time, the second law of thermodynamics says, the entropy of an isolated system can increase, but not decrease. In other words, what we measure is the expansion of the ever-present universe & moment around us, & because we are conscious of that we equate that to "time."

Why am I talking about this in a Fitness Self - Help book? Because essentially we constantly put off what needs to be considered a priority for the sake of doing it another "time" Think about the last time you wanted to work out, but allowed minor friction to get in the way for example; those emails you don't really need to do right now but want to get out of the way. Or my favorite, knowing you need to make some changes to your nutrition & opposed to starting after the bad breakfast or bad lunch you say, "I'll start tomorrow." & continue on with dismantling that burger, "alley-ooping" countless cheese fries with your partner as you Netflix & Chill. With everything we discussed in this chapter, essentially there is no time, only change. So really, you're perpetuating the problem, shoveling it off ironically into another "time" in life.

This used to be me. I used to have minor nutritional "infractions" during my day, & as opposed to saying to myself "I can still make some good choices" I willingly allowed myself to do the ones I specifically know will hinder my progress. In the grand scheme of things, if we want to be great (no matter what form that takes) we must realize the "time" to act is now. All we really have in essence is the present moment allotted to us & the decisions we make in that space. My brother used to tell me growing up, "the summer will be here whether you're ready or not." Although it was tagged to something seemingly trivial, there is a lot of weight to those words if you dissect the context.

Whether you're working towards your ideal or sitting solemnly in the dumps, "time" will pass. In those repeated moments of action, day in - day out the time will come where either all the hard work you put in finally paid off or you yielded nothing because of your inconsistency. I used to have (still do from time to time) clients complain to me that they weren't making the progress they would like to see. When this happens, I don't get defensive, I allow the client to tell me what I'm doing right or wrong & what I can do to change up a little bit. However, I always ask similar questions as well so we can get to a happy medium of understanding. One question I would always ask is "Do you do the workouts (homework) I sent you to do 3 times a week?" More often than not I get "I could only do 1 session because I had no time." To that I always firmly reply with "Hogwash."

We have the time for the things we make a priority. It's not even real! So, what is the difference between doing something later, as opposed to doing something the moment it was previously scheduled? If the answer is because you didn't feel motivated, then there is a reality check in order. I truly don't believe our ancestors ever did anything because they felt like it or was waiting to be picked up by the wings of motivation. You're more likely to never complete the task if you consistently put it off, & things tend to escalate very quickly if unchecked. One day you're not working out & eating against your nutritional goals, next day you're 20lbs plus & de-conditioned. Life comes at you fast. We can all benefit from being more disciplined. How you do one thing is how you do everything, who you choose to be & what you do in those moments determines your trajectory, whether that be in regard to fitness or elsewhere. The time to start is always now.

 The worst feeling, we can feel is regret. Regret for the things we may have done to others is one of them, depending what kind of lifestyle you live. However, the greatest regret comes from the things we didn't do. Ever have those moments when you're alone, sitting & reflecting on the movie that is your life? As you take account of your actions you always think of things you've done, but we always stumbled towards the realm of "what if?" One example that comes to mind from my personal life is the time of my senior year in high school. I had this biggest crush on this girl (who shall remain nameless) for years & she never knew, even though we were great friends.

 The relationship was platonic & out of my fear of potentially ruining the relationship I never acted on it. 'til this day I still think about what could've been. Maybe not with such intense seething pain of not acting upon my desires at time, willing to risk it all in the name of love, but rather a chance to play a film I will never experience. In a way that is so poetic yet heartbreaking. If our lives truly are movies, let us play the role of the courageous character, willingly to brave the elements & explore what truly life has to offer & become the greatest of ideals without hindrance. Love your movie. Be the lead actor or actress & take charge of your life. Because before you know it the credits *will* be rolling.

 One of my ultimate fears is laying on my death bed with or without my loved ones, thinking "wow I wonder what would've happened if I did what I really wanted." Only to know in seconds I now have to make peace with the fact I will never open my eyes again. This is why I work hard on my own endeavors. The fear of dying and leaving it all on the table.

 What's a fear of yours that's holding you back from living one of the greatest lives ever, through your eyes?

Chapter 8 - Remember your why

What is your why? Seriously. Why do you do the things you do? There may not be any esoteric, noble reason for the things you do but have you ever asked yourself "why am I doing this?" We humans act on impulse when we're not cognizant of it. Arguments showcase this perfectly. When we're not paying attention & in the heat of it all, we can explode with anger, saying this we didn't mean to say. Oftentimes we lack the ability to step back & take into account our emotions & someone else's.

But what about when it comes to everyday nature? Take a family size bag of chips for example. You sit there with the bag watching the moving, usually starting with a single chip. Before you know it, here you are with the 3/4th's of the bag already making its way past your digestive tract. To make things worse, you were just starting out your new diet today & everything was working out so well.

What happened here? Much like overspending, when we don't take into account what we're doing we tend to go overboard. This isn't to say count out everything you eat & be as specific as possible, down to the very micronutrient. However, ask yourself "what strategies can I implement to make sure I don't go overboard?" Having a plan works but having a plan for when things can go wrong is different. Just like Batman, we all could use a contingency plan or two in our battle against the bulge. How to calculate your shortcomings will greatly vary the rate of success of whatever you're doing.

When I was younger my mother rarely bought snacks into the house. I thought she hated us. My grandmother took absolutely advantage of this & played the role of a saint & candy smuggler, pedaling me Hershey Kisses in the middle of church sermons. That woman knew what she was doing. She was my contingency plan for the lack of snacks in the house. It was awesome, & I paid dearly for it by becoming 170lbs at 11 years old, & on my way to becoming heavier as time went on. As I got older & started living on my own, I noticed during my own food shopping I wouldn't buy snacks either. As children naturally we do what parents do, not what we're told so seeing my mom buy vegetables & healthy foods gave me the information & know how in order to live a healthy lifestyle as I got older.

This was a contingency plan perfectly in plain sight. The idea is absolutely perfect. Not having snacks in the house means you have to literally go out of your way to go get them. In this case the further you live the better, because this will eventually quell the motivation you have burning from within for those Sweet & Spicy Doritos. Unless you live in NYC where there is a bodega every 150ft from each other. But the fact remains the same, if it is out of sight, it's out of mind. Just like your ex. Or maybe not now, now that I've just mentioned it.

I've learned that with a lot of clients, some have watched others live with bad habits, replicate it in their own fashion & when they want to make a change, they fall prey to their old ways, starting the cycle again. Sometimes we still have to make the conscious jump of implementing new changes, instead of just wanting them internally. When we make this jump successfully, our outward actions match our inner desires making us that much more likely to succeed. The better you're at making the things you want (that are "bad" for you) harder to access, the more discipline you'll have when it comes to diet & exercise.

Growing up I hated how my mother raised me, in a way. Everything had to be tidy, things kept in order, clothes done, homework done. My mother was never in the military, but she kept & ran a tight ship in that household. Now that I live on my own, I can't imagine life any other way & guiltily I admit, sometimes when I am in someone's home, I scan the area for miscellaneous items. Not judging, but my mind is so conditioned to put things away I sometimes rearrange someone else's things if it seems un-orderly. Something I'm still working on.

Our environment at a very early age dictates the type of person we become, & society will agree. So much so that the phrase "that's just the way I am" or "that's just the way it is" is constantly being thrown around in defiance to change. I agree sometimes people can be pushy & demanding, trying to force their ideals on you. But to be fair, exclaiming "that's just the way it is!" as a response to something you did or something that happened to you, & not taking or making the opportunity to make it right isn't fair either. Mainly it's unfair to you. You rob your own self of the opportunity to turn things around. Have you ever asked yourself why?

When we exclaim these words, we accept the fact that we believe we cannot overcome our circumstances. Words certainly do have power, especially within the person that says them. However, it is the action & the way in which we essentially prime our minds to be aware of the opportunities we lack, or the opportunities around us. We defeat ourselves before we ever step on the battlefield. Sometimes my clients would mention that they just had to stop & get something to eat otherwise they would "pass out" or simply needed to eat something in the meantime.

These urges are natural to succumb too. The body is primed for comfort, but not cognizant of automatically turning you away from what's not ideal so it is entirely up to you to make a firm conscious decision to make a change. It doesn't have to be as daunting as it may seem to be, & your changes don't have to be instant. We want to make changes that stick for the long haul. Your life can potentially be a long one. What you want it to be like depends on your ability to separate what you want now for the future, work hard without seeing the pay off so soon, having faith that everything will work out in the end.

There will be times where things seem tough, like you haven't made any progress & everything you've been doing has been a waste of time. We play cruel jokes on ourselves by not giving ourselves the just do props we deserve. Effort should only be measured to what you've tried in the past, & every day is a chance to do it better or at the very least "break even." These are incredible times to figure out or remember your why. Why do you do what you do? What's the fire that keeps you going when things get tough.

For me that's my mother. Losing both of my brothers brought us closer together & in a way has renewed my hopes for a brighter tomorrow. Seeing her smile is a great feeling, & her knowing that I'm striving to get better every day makes her proud & myself as well. Things weren't always like this though. We never spoke much, primarily because we didn't see eye to eye on many things growing up. I was truly a rebel & we both were stubborn individuals, never liking to admit when we were wrong. However, when both of my brothers passed it was almost as if all this armor came down & we both came to the realization that indeed life is short & better to make the most of it as opposed to regretting things were different.

The reality is our relationship needed a lot of work & we needed to be honest with ourselves. Years of burying our differences in the sea of silence quickly came back to shore when we spoke more consistently. This time around we were able to talk like adults. Both growing from our perspectives & being able to create a healthier relationship dynamic, no longer based on commands & responses. Our dialogue is more of the friend variety, something I never thought I would see growing up. I'm glad it happened. Death has taught me that you never know when people will go, so it's best to settle differences & get along in the meantime, we can all make the world a better place that way.

Now when I wake up, I have a mission. Making my mom, but my family proud as well. Ethereal or not. Mix that with a little bit of my fear of failure & I have a nice motivation cocktail to start my day. If we must be afraid of something, may it be the fear of becoming greater than what we are, opposed to being afraid of not being able to change. I believe that is where we get our stubbornness from. The logic behind it, when I think of it is "well why would anyone want to try something new if they feel they would fail every time?"

Frankly, I agree. If I were to feel like I was not good at anything I try, I wouldn't try either. But what if you haven't really tried? How many times have you "attempted" things half-heartedly, only to be disappointed to miss the mark? Of course, you were going to miss, you didn't try at all! This may sound harsh, who am I to determine the capacity of someone else's exertion? But it does have some merit. Your ceilings are made of glass. They were meant to be shattered.

Behind all the negative thoughts, doubts, bullies, bad memories, moments, photos etc., lies something within you, potential! You have a great ability to change your life for the better, make the changes you wish so, without falling off weeks or months from the time you start. We have to do an honest appraisal of where we are in relation to our goals, & consciously, gradually make these changes that will stay the course, bringing us closer inline to them. This is a lifestyle change, not a quick fix so it pays to do your due diligence.

What areas do you seem to be struggling with the most? If it's nutrition, consider "dieting" your house. Basically, you'd no longer consume & get rid of the snacks you have at the time being. You may be reading that sentence again thinking I'm crazy for saying throw out new food. You don't necessarily have to throw them out, you could opt to give the food away so long as the snacks are out of the house for the time allotted. That can help encourage you to keep going for longer time periods without or quitting altogether. Either of which is a win – win.

What about fitness? How can you tailor it to work better for you? Consider your new workout program which we created in the previous chapter. How can you tweak the time of, or repetitions of each exercise to align with your goals? Sometimes the smallest tweaks give the biggest payoff. Don't overlook the things you can control even if they appear menial. If you're willing to have a hands-on approach with your fitness you get the opportunity to build a good foundation of fitness which can set, you up for a lifetime. When you learn the fundamentals, it allows for total creativity in a way that will keep you progressing through your exercises & enjoying them. They say knowledge is power, but it is also confidence. Confident that you are up to the task at hand & can complete it efficiently. This is self-efficacy, tried & true.

Chapter 9 - A better me starts with a better you

   Picture this; It's been two years since you first started with your workout program. You now workout 5 - 6 days a week, & you have found a nutritional concept that works for both you & your goals. You feel great! Clothes are no longer a problem. You finally feel confident in the things you wear, & that confidence can be seen for miles! Breathing as you walk upstairs is much easier, you enjoy going for hikes now & have even made new friends to keep up with your new hobby. You're much more productive at work, so much so your boss decides to give you a promotion after your review. People can see the energy that now radiates off of you & for the first time in a while things feel great.

   You walk into the coffee shop; you get your favorite brew & you're ready for the next wave of emails inbound to your inbox. You professionally message, reply & book everything that needs to be marked on that calendar, your presentation is on point & the speech has been rehearsed so many times you can do it with your eyes closed. You're on top of the world, baby. Then it happens, your ex walks in. Or maybe your crush. Either way, whoever is capable of sinking your heart enters the room. You stare blankly, thinking you've seen a ghost. You two make eye contact, but they're smiling?

   They walk over to you surprisingly happy. They may be excited to share what's been going on with them but to your own surprise the first thing that comes out of their mouth is "Hey (insert name here)! Wow, you look incredible. How'd you do it?" You explain, you created your own workout program & stuck to it, loved the results & kept going. Not only are they impressed they even ask you if you could help them. That's when this all comes around full circle.

   You realize all that hard work finally did pay off, not only on the inside but the outside as well. You may have noticed you've gained mental strength as well as physical strength! But best of all, not only do you have the ability to change your life (which you always had), now you have a skill that if cultivated through proper certifications you can help make an impact on other people's lives as well! You have proverbially learned how to fish; now - can you now help others?

   I think the best part of fitness is how influential you could be to someone. I feel fulfilled knowing that I'm helping other people steer towards better lifestyle choices in order to help them keep doing what they love in the first place. When I think back to my own journey, I remember the humble beginnings in which I got my first feel as a coach. It was a long journey, & one that keeps going. That's the mind-bending part of it all. I may be able to write a book on this material myself, but I am also constantly learning, trying new things & weeding out the ones that do not. It's a precarious position of teacher & student, one that can shift easily as new information is discovered.

The fitness industry is inherently dying in some respects. As today's marketing machines become more influencer based it becomes more about doing something that works for the ideal body, which may not be yours. How does that work? I see tons of these "Look Like XYZ" person programs only 12 weeks for an exorbitant number that doesn't reflect the value of the program offered. It's easy to see why as more information comes out people are getting more confused, & others are capitalizing on the uneducated in regard to this topic.

When I started out in fitness, I made my own workouts by looking them up. Now everyone looks to someone else to make a program for them, which is fine - this is what gives people jobs & stimulates the economy. However, what about when that person is gone, or you are no longer able to afford to keep up with the Joneses, letting go of your Tier 3 Equinox trainer? Do you revert to having no muscle again? Do you revert to being out of shape? Absolutely not! You're more likely to stick to spin classes for the rest of your life instead of doing that.

I wanted to give the consumer their power back. All these fitness services are great (including my own) but what about creating something you like to do for a change? Fitness allows for freedom & I think if you're unsure of making your own program you can never truly discover fitness for yourself but also it makes the programs you do routine. I enjoy doing a different workout after weeks of doing my own because I get to come back to the drawing board & add something different. The more exercises I'm able to perform confidently I can translate to my clients as well, also enhancing their knowledge, while strengthening my own. But when you constantly go to a Class Pass session with the same instructor over & over again, things get routine & stale - fast.

When you are able to make your own program, essentially, you're able to take the training wheels off and pursue more challenging exercises & styles. This I would say is true freedom. When you now come across these new movements & techniques, you'll understand them better & use them more efficiently because you already know the breakdown of certain exercises because you know their regression.

We all want change. Whether that be with our own lives or on the global stage, we are all aware that something needs to be done. Sometimes we scream these with vigor from the mountain tops, but I ask in the midst of all the rage & angst, what if we change ourselves first? Would the world around us then start to change? This sounds like it will be a collective effort, but I think it's possible. We need to be keen & zero in on our moments of appraisal if we expect change from society at large.

Change, physical or mental, or both is essential to human development. Man, unless forced by trauma does not mentally stay the knowledge & perception level of an infant. As the human grows so does the intellect, opinions & all the little quirks that make us, us. That doesn't mean we always move with the best intentions & are rather hypocritical in nature when we scrutinize something. But what if the tables were turned? What if we are as crucial to ourselves as we are with other people? Could we see a wave of accountability begin to crop up throughout the country?

The hallmark of a good leader is one that can lead by example. The good ole monkey see, monkey do. When we see people that seem like they have it all figured out, what do they look like? High energy, calm, serene, kind, full of personality. They seem utterly unshakable & unfazed, two characteristics that seem to be dwindling in today's society, but largely sought after. These feelings are contagious, along with motivating as well.

When I was 13, I started going to the barbershop alone. One particular Saturday I was walking to the shop, when I noticed a brand new (at the time) 2007 BMW 750Li. My jaw dropped when I saw this thing, & I knew I had to meet the owner of the vehicle. When I entered, I noticed an older gentleman sitting off to the side, with the only chair available next to him I sat down. Seeing the car magazine as I approached the table, I figured I could read these magazines in the meantime while I waited for my haircut.

The older gentlemen had started a conversation with another gentlemen about cars, the car in question was the very own 750Li I saw outside, & the owner just so happened to be sitting right next to me. I chimed in with my very limited car knowledge & was accepted into the conversation but only briefly. When I asked him how he got to the level of where he was at the time, he said something to me I will never forget. "If you do what is hard, life will be easy. If you do what is easy, life will be hard." Those words stuck with me always & have been a part of my motivation mantra ever since.

We all want to be the one that has it all figured out. But how much easier is it to do what's comfortable at the time. We all want the "God" body that you see grace the magazines & movie screens, but how much easier is it to have that beer with your friends? To take the temporary pleasures over the delayed gratification you know is going to be 10,000x better is often due to conditioning, how we see ourselves & our self-efficacy towards completing the objective at hand.

 Once you get over that hill, have defeated your "dragons" & have now become a small-town inspiration to everyone you know, what's next? The journey now takes on different paths, what do you want to be? You may have new dreams & aspirations after your newfound weight-loss success. Whatever avenue you choose to continue fueling your fitness journey remember two things. The first one being of which you need to be consistent, always. Remember entropy? One can only expand through time, so there are absolutely no regressions allowed. Forever forward, in turn lighting the way for others that come across your shining light. The second of which is to remember to give back in some form.

 The world needs light. The world needs love. It wasn't until I felt I was at my absolute best that I was able to pour more energy into other people. If we ourselves cannot be selfish with our goals, understanding that if we take care of ourselves better, we can take care of other people better, we can't actually help people! This isn't to say you have to be on the ground doing some volunteer work, but here's an example. When you feel your worst are, you're more likely, or less likely to compliment someone? Of course, less likely. However, if you feel, look & even smell great, your positive vibes will radiate to others around you & you will be handing out compliments like Oprah.

 Compliments are one of the best ways you can lighten up someone's day, & they don't cost a thing. Completely free! If us humans are here to connect & uplift one another, experience what this universe has to offer & make an impact along the way, we owe it to ourselves to have better bodies to handle such a tall order. When you're feeling your best, your light shines through you to other people & they take on that energy. If we can cultivate love, happiness, & understanding from developing ourselves, how much more peace can we experience within the world? If we want to change the world, the change must come from within, and translate throughout.

Chapter 10 - Closing Curtain

 I, like you, have fears. What keeps me up at night are the fears that my mother might pass away before I really accomplish my most ambitious goals. I'm also afraid that I may die before I accomplish my biggest goals & aspirations. Although I'm still young I am absolutely terrified of wasting time so to speak. Not that I am constantly in a rush, but sometimes I get this feeling that makes me feel like leisure time shouldn't be had just yet. I think I've taken the mantra "one more" too closely to heart. This is something that I am working on. So, in some ways my fear has a pro & con, the fear of not accomplishing my most ambitious goals keeps me focused in a timely manner in an effort to reach them within the time allotted. The downside is my neuroticism may kick in thus affecting my ability to overexert myself in time.

 This is how all our fears work. They have a litany of pros & cons, making it our job to regulate what we can & let go of the things we can't control. Once we're able to see that, that's when the changes take place & we are then able to make the changes necessary to overcome what we are facing. Using fear, as a tool it becomes the fuel you need to get over the obstacle in your path. However, when fear is left unregulated it takes hold of all logical processing rendering you vulnerable to your situation. The goal here is to manage what you can & shirk the responsibility of anything you cannot. What you cannot change is not up to you to change ultimately. This is why we suffer! Because we feel the need to still bear emotional attachments to things we ultimately cannot change, whether those attachments have good intentions or not.

 It's been nearly 10 years since my brother Didier has passed. Although my brother Jerry also passed away, I do not have as much survival guilt as I do with my brother Dj. Survivor's guilt can often be described as ones feeling guilty for surviving a traumatic event, while the other did not. It's a feeling unlike anything I ever experienced. A wave of guilt came over me during those years, I felt like I should have been with him that day & ultimately let him down. In the worst way possible at that. It was a lot for my 17-year-old mind to take in at that time, so I had kept to myself & stayed inside, hidden away from everyone in my attic alone in my room with my brothers 5 feet apart from mine. Waiting for him to come home.

 I still think of him until this day, & how could I couldn't? That was my brother after all. The same kid that used to pick me up when I was 5 wrestling with me, I was now laying to rest. My heart broke into a million fragments that day, & the innocence I had was surely gone. The kid in me died that day & never came back. I was different, for good. But at the time, I didn't think it was for the good. I had spent the next couple of years hating everything. Mad at the world for what had happened. Finally coming to my senses & going back to the gym things started to make sense.

The conclusion I came to in those years was that I could no longer be sad for what happened because eventually the same thing is going to happen to me. In fact, the same thing will happen to you as well, sorry if you were misinformed. The reaper comes for us all, in many forms. Let's just pray the passing is peaceful. With that said, I had decided that I was going to live life on my terms & how I wanted from that point forward, doing things like becoming a Personal Trainer & making music as well. Even going so far as opening up for Method Man & Redman at Star-land Ballroom. I or we rather, don't know when our time is up, so why play it safe? Why not start that project you've always wanted? Why not work for the body you want & see how far you can go with it? Why live by any boundaries if one day we will have none as ethereal elements of the world?

Humans as a species have overcome many obstacles, you as an individual has as well. What makes us so driven is our self-efficacy. When we know we can do something we are more motivated to try. This goes for every single person that has achieved something great. They believed in themselves. If the faith of a mustard is all that is necessary, how much more faith & focus can you have when you have the tools, the know how & the confidence to match? There is no telling what you are capable of in the world so long as you are willingly to try. I admire Ralph Waldo Emerson's belief in self-reliance for that reason. Emerson states that self-reliance & the ability to make the best choice comes from the individual & the individual only.

The ability to assume responsibility is one of the hardest skills to acquire. This entails that every decision you make, you take full responsibility for regardless of the outcome. When you know in your heart the decision you make is best for you, you must take action to back that choice. Then & only then will you find what you are truly made of. In a society constantly telling you to conform, the voice inside our head voicing our truest desire is dwindling over time. Eventually we find ourselves working a job we hate, doing things we don't really like & potentially even in a relationship that truly doesn't fulfill us. Here I ask, what is the point of living a life you don't like if only to please other people?

What a lie we tell ourselves that we have to do certain things to make people happy. This isn't me trying to disrupt the nuclear family in any way, but much like Emerson I believe in self-reliance as well. To allow other people to make decisions for us, strips us of our true freedom & ultimately our truest self. What a worse way to end it all? On your deathbed with the ghost of what could've been if you only had followed your dreams.

You must be informed to make those choices, which is partly why I wanted to write this book. Giving the reader the power back so to speak. With a lot of information out on the internet, I've taken that & a decade of professional - personal experience into a no frills straight to the point book that helps you create a 12-week workout program, & a brief overview on nutrition. However, this doesn't mean you should listen to me. Yes, there are fundamentals you must follow which are addressed in this book, but the reality is, if learning the information has motivated you to get started, take the next step & start doing some research on your own! Discover what makes you tick when it comes to fitness.

You may like running, yoga, boxing, powerlifting you name it. Whatever you come across in your research, dare to challenge it by doing it yourself & take notes. The more you practice treating yourself as the "test subject" the more informed you become on the matter. Please note that you should not take this advice too far & do something that is way too far out of your scope. Remember Bambi, baby step before you run.

Finally knowing where you're going brings this all together. When you have the tools, the skills, & the know-how, you just need some direction. Making your weight loss goal a S.M.A.R.T. goal will help you stay on track & set attainable goals in the window you have given yourself. S.M.A.R.T. stands for "specific, measurable, attainable, relevant & time bound. Use this building criteria for your goals & check back with it frequently to make sure you're on task & up to date. When you write your goals, you're more likely to achieve them in general, but S.M.A.R.T. goals create the laser - like focus criteria needed to ensure success. Consider using them not just for fitness, but for other areas in your life as well.

If you have read up until this point, I want to say thank you. Thank you for being the reason I wrote this book. I may never meet you, but I hope these words have sparked the imagination from within you & has given you the tools necessary to get started changing your life. We've learned the major movement planes, different dieting strategies, & how to put together a workout program including the reps & sets. I am forever thankful to my brother Didier for introducing me to the gym world. Fitness & reading have saved my life more times than I really know, so it only felt right to write a book about the subject. Fitness also gave me some of the best memories with my brothers I will ever have, & for that I am thankful. My brother used to jog with me from time to time & we would always crack jokes while running, eventually slowing down to just walking. They were the best hangout sessions I ever had with anyone; we would always have great conversations & now they are memories I can cherish for as long as I'm here.

When I think of the grand scheme of life, I often wonder why things happen the way they do. So many times, in my life I had wished I could go back in time to say goodbye one more time, or even spend one more day, but life is not designed that way. This is a movie with no fast forward or rewind, simply play. A movie that sometimes is a nightmare, sometimes is too good to be true. But just about all of the time, the movie is ours. We may not notice; we may live in the shadow of someone else, but we can always change roles.

Life has plenty of solum moments, but it is because of those very moments that the sun shining on a beautiful day can bring you to tears by its simplistic beauty. Seeing people live life & enjoy themselves is the motivation that keeps me going. I love the idea of life & what it has to offer, & it is my hope that everyone in life can see the simple things for the beauty they possess, the finer things for the enrichment they provide & appreciate one another because we can truly change one another's lives.

Before my brother Jerry passed away, we had talked about the future & what we wanted to achieve. Jerry had NFL dreams when he was younger but because of injuries & life circumstances he never went pro. But he played semi pro until his passing. He was sad that he was unable to play anymore because he was developing blood clots, but I tried to encourage him & let him know that with his skills he could be a coach. He tried but the offer fell through, more sadness ensued. I again tried to encourage him, but it seemed like it was almost all but hopeless. When I would FaceTime him, I would notice the light in his eyes were gone, the sign of a man who was already dead way before his body had ceased to function. He was a shell of his former self.

I'll never forget that last conversation. I told him that I was going to have a Condo in California, & a list of other future items I had waiting for me. He encouraged me to keep working hard but reminded me about how hard life was, and proceeded to let me know that it was okay if I failed. I realized instantly in that moment he had a fixed mindset. But that was brother, so I replied back "I guess we'll find out when I'm your age." in the most condescending tone. Unfortunately, however, we were never able to have that conversation as he died just a couple months later in a car crash. At 36 years old, my second & last brother I had on Earth passed away. Some days I feel like I am truly lonely in this world, but I am glad I've been able to turn my negatives into positives. I end this book on a somber yet motivating tone;

Be that as it may, whether alone or with an army at my side, I will still overcome any & all obstacles. YOU WILL as well. As my contribution to the world, I give this book in hopes that you will be inspired to live life on your terms. Take back your power. You can become whatever your heart desires so long as you can put in the work.

The road may be long & arduous, but there will come a time where people will see you one day & ask "how did you do it?" You'll tell them you took up the responsibility to take your fitness, and your life seriously by doing your own research & putting in the time & effort. In that moment you will have inspired someone to start their own journey, & the cycle continues. You never know when & where you can impact someone's life, & it all starts by changing your own.

Merci et bénissez-vous.